TIPS PREGNANT WOMEN SHOULD FOLLOW

For a Healthy Pregnancy And Safe Delivery

ROSE JOHN JAMES

TABLE OF CONTENT

CHAPTER 1

FIRST TIME PREGNANCY

Being pregnant is a joyous time that often motivates women to lead better lifestyles and, if necessary, strive for a healthy body weight. Here are some suggestions for making your nutrition and exercise habits better both throughout pregnancy and after giving birth.

These suggestions might be helpful even if you are not pregnant but are considering becoming a parent. Making adjustments now will allow you to adapt to new lifestyle patterns. You'll provide your child with the finest possible start in life and set an example of good health for the whole family.

Before you can take care of your new baby, you need to take care of yourself and your unborn child. There's a lot of advice out there.

- Exercise consistently

It's difficult to have a kid, both physically and psychologically. Exercise often to ward against the discomfort and emotional fluctuations that accompany pregnancy.

- Low-impact exercise may enhance your mood, boost circulation, and relieve back discomfort. In order to prepare for labor, it will help strengthen your muscles and ligaments.

- Swimming and walking are two excellent activities that minimize the impact on your body. Prenatal yoga helps with restlessness, hip opening, stress relief, and boosts conception rates.

- Heavy weightlifting and strenuous aerobic activities may be more harmful than beneficial.

- Drink a lot of water First-time mothers need more water than usual since it is incorporated into the amniotic fluid that surrounds the developing fetus. Low fluid levels may cause miscarriage, birth abnormalities, and difficult childbirth.

Since you require more than usual while pregnant, you might quickly get dehydrated. To keep hydrated, it is advised that you consume at least 10 cups of 8 ounces of liquid each day.

Additionally, drinking adequate water will reduce joint swelling and remove toxins from your system.

- Utilize naps

It's typical to feel tired, particularly in the first trimester. Your body is undergoing hormonal changes that will have an impact on how much energy you have.

- Spend some time right now getting some rest and allowing your body to unwind. You won't have as much time to relax after the kid is delivered. Your sleep routine will be irregular and incomplete.

- Therefore, indulge yourself to a sleep in the afternoon to recharge and lessen the strain of work and home life on your child.

- It's also critical to get the appropriate quantity of sleep at night. It will become harder to sleep at night as your pregnancy goes on. You'll struggle to find a comfortable position for your_bump and often need the restroom.

- Your hips will be in alignment if you use a cushion, relieving strain on your back and pelvis.

- Maternity Massage

Make an appointment for a skilled prenatal massage before giving birth.

- Lower back discomfort, which may be dangerous throughout your pregnancy, is treated with a low-impact massage. Additionally, it will improve circulation and reduce swelling-causing irritation.

- At the beginning of your first trimester, stay away from massages. Since there is a larger probability of miscarriage during this period, the majority of practitioners won't accept women. After then, you may get a message at any moment until your due date.

- Establish a birth plan

When your kid is born, you start off as a mother. You want to make this occasion memorable and secure. Making a birth plan is crucial for this reason.

- Before heeding any advise from friends and relatives, do your own web study about your possibilities. Since this is your choice, you should have an objective understanding of the various delivery options.

You have more options than just where you will be. A few other choices include having a water delivery, getting an epidural, or delaying the cord clamping.

- Buy something

Get ready those necessary and adorable newborn goods to celebrate the arrival of your bundle of joy.

With a crib, changing table, rocking chair, and dresser, you can set up the nursery. Additionally, choose a lively color for the walls and window decals that your youngster will appreciate.

Although dressing your kid is enjoyable, it also involves a lot of preparation. When your baby has a growth spurt, you don't want to be without clothing. Consider purchasing a size larger than their present age. Only purchase a few newborn outfits since they won't last very long.

Additionally, you should pick cloth or reusable inserts or diaper brands. Disposable diapers are ideal for babies since you will be changing them often. You could change to a more environmentally friendly alternative as they age.

Blankets, bibs, bottles, and some beginner toys are important items to remember.

You may get ready for your new addition physically and psychologically with the aid of these things.

CHAPTER 2

WHY A HEALTHY DIET IS BENEFICIAL FOR MOM AND BABY

Generally speaking, eating well has a lot of advantages. A healthy diet gives a woman several benefits, like increased stamina, a better immune system, and a lower chance of illness, to mention a few. Because they are also eating for the health of their unborn child when they are pregnant, pregnant women need to be extra cautious about what they consume. When a pregnant woman eats healthily, she lowers her risk of issues including anemia, low birth weight, and birth abnormalities. Healthy eating might also lessen uncomfortable pregnancy symptoms! The advantages of a good pregnancy diet are listed below.

- **Less complexity**

Although it might be challenging, resisting undesirable pregnancy cravings is ultimately beneficial for the wellbeing of both you and your unborn child. You can be at risk for issues including gestational diabetes, anemia, urinary tract infections, and the delivery of a child with birth abnormalities if you don't follow a balanced diet. It's never a bad thing, but healthy eating throughout pregnancy may help make labor and delivery easier!

- **Enhanced Energy**

For the majority of women, feeling so exhausted during pregnancy that they can hardly move is extremely typical. No matter what you do, exhaustion may often be difficult to manage, particularly in the first few weeks when your body is going through a lot of hormonal changes. Your energy levels will be maintained by consuming a healthy meal and doing so every 3 to 4 hours. It's vital to keep in mind that your iron needs should be doubled throughout pregnancy in order to support your larger blood volume and encourage the fetus's ability to store iron.

- **Positive fetal development**

A healthy diet is just what your kid needs to develop properly. You should try to consume at least 300 more calories each day than usual. You don't want to overdo it, either, since that might result in issues like preeclampsia and gestational diabetes. A healthy newborn needs a variety of vitamins and minerals, including but not limited to calcium, folic acid, vitamin C, vitamin A, fiber, fruits, vegetables, whole grains, and enough protein and fat.

- **Better Sleep**

During your pregnancy, a lot of things might keep you awake at night, including nausea, many toilet trips in the middle of the night, or aches and pains! Your beauty sleep will undoubtedly benefit from eating regular, substantial meals and abstaining from excessive coffee. Iron, calcium, and vitamin

B are among the vitamins and minerals required during pregnancy that help promote restful sleep.

- **Lower Chance of Being ill**

Women who are pregnant are more prone to contracting certain illnesses, such as the flu. This may be avoided with a balanced diet and plenty of sleep. Although a simple cold won't likely harm your unborn child, experiencing pregnancy symptoms is unpleasant enough without adding sickness to the mix. It's best to try to be healthy in general!

CHAPTER 3

TIPS FOR PREGNANT WOMEN

- You need a lot of protein, good fats, and additional amounts of a few vitamins and minerals when pregnant (such as folic acid, iron, and calcium). See our list of the vitamins and minerals you need to help your child develop.
- Pregnancy does not need increased calorie intake. You don't need extra calories throughout the first trimester if you begin the pregnancy at a healthy weight. In the second and third trimesters, you'll need an additional 340 and 450 calories each day, respectively. Learn more about weight growth during pregnancy.
- Certain meals might be harmful to you during pregnancy. Find out what to avoid. (During pregnancy, you'll also need to stop drinking alcohol and cut down on caffeine.)

- The best pregnant snacks are healthy ones! Reduce your use of processed meals, packaged foods, and sugary sweets while picking snacks that help you achieve your nutritional requirements.
- Try eating small, frequent meals throughout the day if eating full-size meals is difficult due to nausea, food aversions, heartburn, or indigestion. You won't have as much room in your body for large meals as your pregnancy goes on since your baby will be crammed into your stomach and other digestive organs.
- Do you need further details? Make a pregnant meal plan to ensure that your diet contains all the nutrients you need.

CHAPTER 4

REAL FOOD FOR PREGNANT WOMAN

Nutritional health is more crucial than ever. Include a variety of fruits, vegetables, nutritious grains, protein-rich meals, and fat-free or low-fat dairy items in your prenatal diet to promote a healthy pregnancy and your baby's growth. Reduce your intake of meals and drinks that are high in salt, saturated fat, and added sugar. Make fruits and vegetables the majority of every meal. And take pleasure in the pregnancy-friendly meals mentioned below!

Eggs

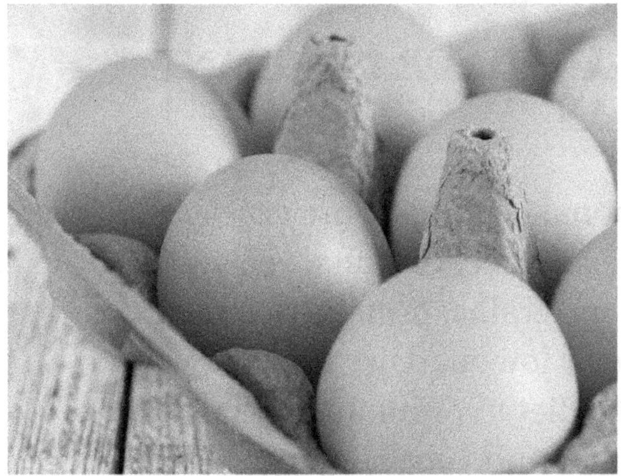

A vital component of your pregnancy diet and a fantastic source of protein are eggs. The building blocks of both your and your baby's cells are the amino acids that make up protein minerals, including choline, are also present in eggs. Choline aids your baby's brain and spinal cord in developing normally and helps avoid certain birth abnormalities; it is mostly found in the yolks, so be sure to eat those.

The components of a frittata are eggs, any vegetables and cheese you happen to have on hand, and cheese. If there are any leftovers, they are ideal for breakfast the next morning.

Recipe: chard, red onion, and feta frittata

Ratatouille recipe with baked eggs

Salmon

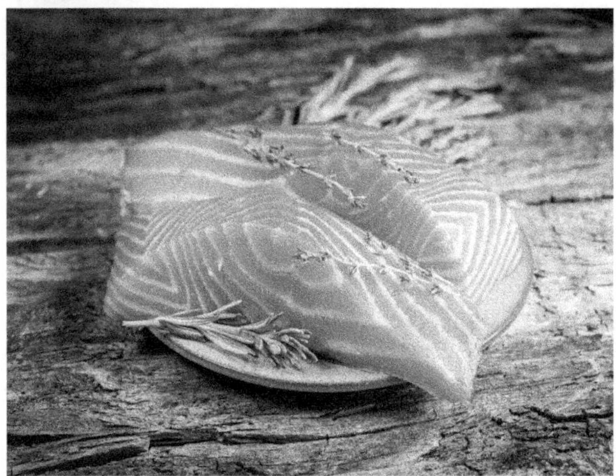

The brain development of your kid depends on omega-3 fatty acids, which may also improve your mood. A particularly excellent source is salmon. The protein and vitamin D in salmon are both essential for your baby's strong bones and teeth.

Salmon is a low-mercury alternative for the 8 to 12 ounces of seafood pregnant women are advised to consume each week, along with herring, trout, anchovies, sardines, and shad. Learn more about eating fish safely while expecting.

Salmon with lentils and leeks, pan-seared

Recipe: BLTs with roasted fish and herbed mayo

Beans

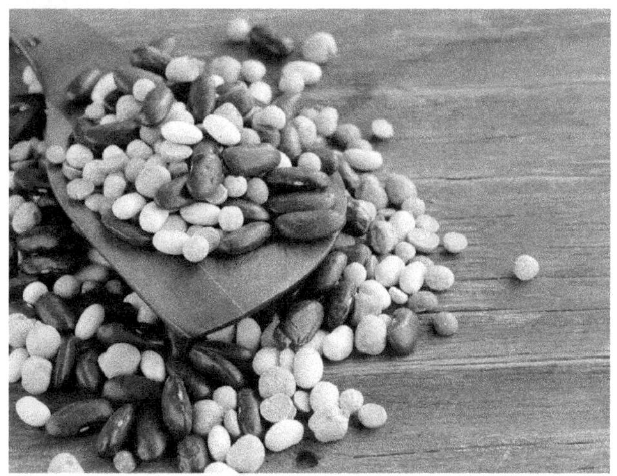

Beans are a strong source of protein and a great supply of iron, folate, potassium, and magnesium. Beans also include legumes like lentils, peas, and peanuts. When you are pregnant, they are all significant.

Beans are an excellent source of fiber, which may prevent and treat the two frequent pregnant aches and pains of hemorrhoids and constipation.

Consider adding edamame, which are cooked soybeans and a fantastic source of vital fatty acids, to salads, soups, or stir-fries. can eat roasted edamame as a snack.

Creamy white beans with bread crumbs, broccolini, and sausage (extra easy, thanks to canned beans)

Stir-fry with broccoli, sugar snap peas, and tofu

Sweet potatoes

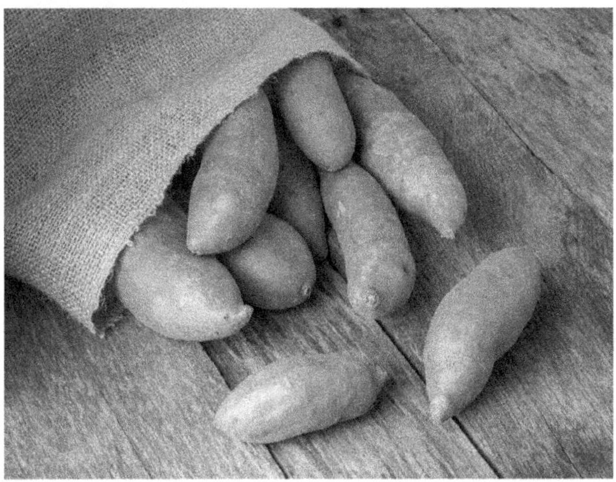

Carotenoids, which are plant pigments that human bodies convert to vitamin A, give sweet potatoes their orange hue. For the development of strong bones, lungs, eyes, and skin in your newborn, vitamin A is essential. This delicious vegetable is also a rich source of fiber, potassium, manganese, vitamin B6 (which may assist during morning sickness), and vitamin C. (especially if you keep the skin on).

Sweet potato and curry-flavored chickpea turnover.

Whole grains

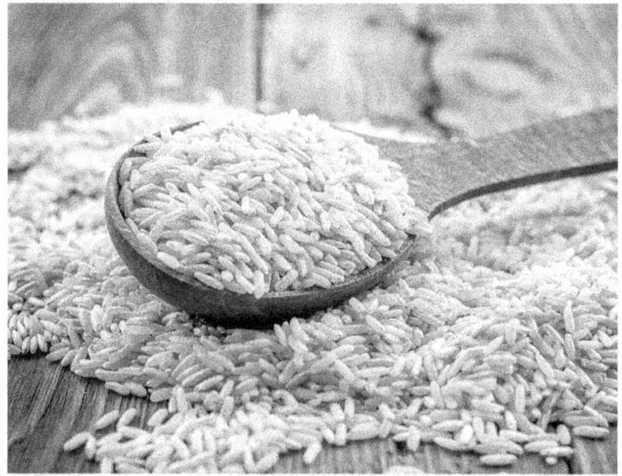

Whole grains are high in fiber and nutrients,including B vitamins, iron, folic acid (if fortified), magnesium, the antioxidant vitamin E, and the mineral selenium. They also contain phytonutrients, plant compounds that protect cells.

Trade white bread for whole grain, and sample different kinds of whole grains – from barley and buckwheat to oats and spelt – in your pregnancy diet.

Recipe: Chicken soup with farro and shiitake mushrooms

Recipe: Quinoa with shrimp, tomato, and avocado

Greek Yogurt

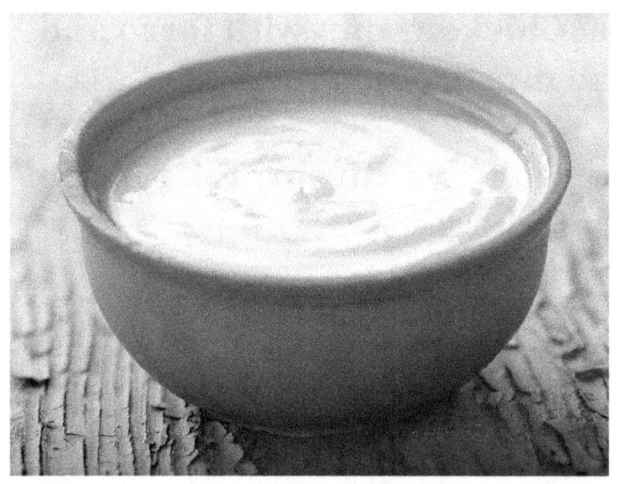

Protein content in Greek yogurt is generally double that of normal yogurt. Probiotics, B vitamins, phosphate, and calcium are also abundant in it. Calcium supports the development of your baby's skeleton and keeps your own bones robust.

Yogurt is a flexible component for breakfast and tastes well in savory recipes as well. Another great method to obtain your daily dose of calcium is by drinking milk.

Cauliflower steaks baked in yogurt with herbs (Note: Roasting this cruciferous vegetable has a reputation for converting critics of cauliflower.)

Honey-yogurt mustard dipping sauce recipe (baked chicken tenders optional)

Honey-yogurt mustard dipping sauce recipe (optional: baked chicken

CHAPTER 5

SAFE EXERCISES FOR PREGNANT WOMEN

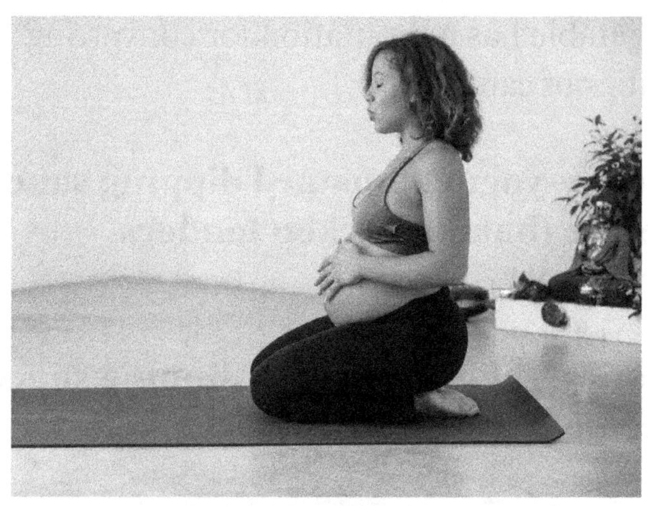

The World Health Organization (WHO) advises pregnant women to engage in at least 150 minutes per week of moderate-intensity aerobic activity.

You don't have to do everything all at once, which is excellent news. You may want to stretch out your physical activity throughout the course of the week. For instance, you might decide to exercise for 30 minutes each day, five days a week. You may also divide it up into smaller time blocks throughout the day. as long as you adhere to the WHO recommendations.

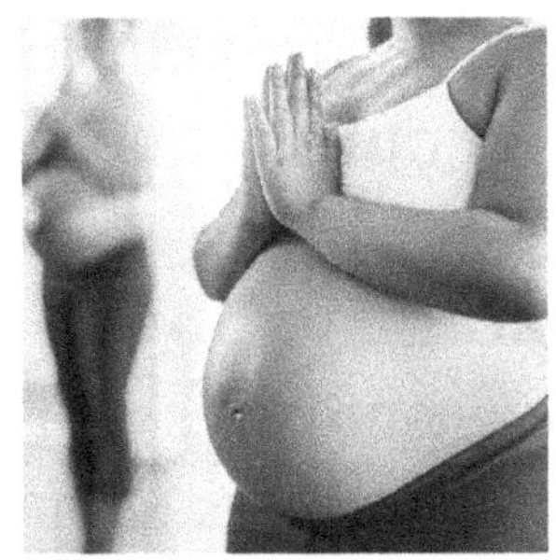

- **Walking**

Start by taking a little walk in the neighborhood. This works every muscle in the body and is gentle on the joints and muscles.

- **Dancing**

It is a terrific method to maintain flexibility and tone your muscles, in addition to allowing you to move your body to your favorite music.

- **Swimming**

The best place to exercise when pregnant is in water since the reduced force of gravity makes you feel lighter. In the water, you may do as many workouts as you choose.

Try swimming if you have low back discomfort during other activities.

- **Exercising Flexibility**

These relax tense muscles and improve back pain. Examples include: cat position, child pose, side stretches, etc.

- **Practice your pelvic floor (Kegel exercises)**

These greatly minimize the possibility of urine leakage both during pregnancy and after delivery by strengthening the pelvic floor muscles.

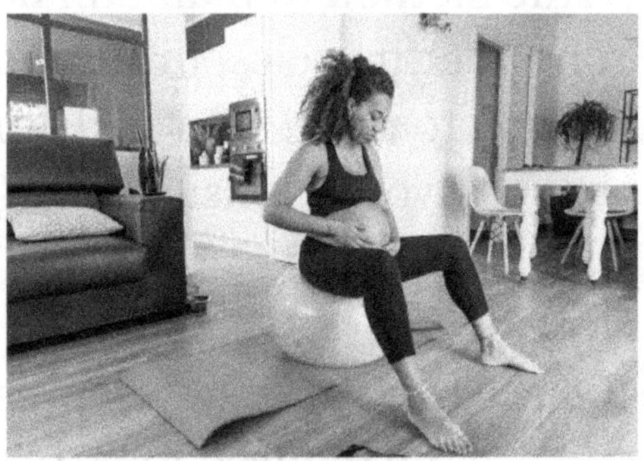

How to execute Kegels

- To prevent any urinary infections, start by emptying your bladder.
- By visualizing yourself peeing and then contracting your muscles to halt the flow of urine or stop the wind from leaving, you may find the correct muscles.
- Five seconds of muscular contraction is followed by five seconds of muscle relaxation.
- Five times in succession, repeat this technique.
- Advance to deeper contractions.
- Attempt not to hold your breath while doing this, and try to relax your abdominal muscles.

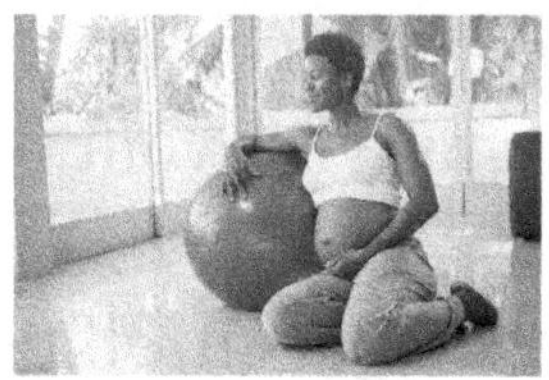

Warning!

Please wait until your doctor has given the all-clear before starting an exercise regimen during pregnancy.

Stop exercising right away and see your doctor if you have faintness, heart palpitations, chest discomfort, contractions, or any odd change in your baby's movements during or after physical exercise.

www.ingramcontent.com/pod-product-compliance
Lightning Source LLC
LaVergne TN
LVHW020538160826
845677LV00015B/4139
9798847435314